SHATTERING THE CHAINS

A journey to break free from depression

HEPHZI PENNS

Matters Of The Heart (MOTH) Publications
00233-245917238

<u>DEDICATION</u>

To all the warriors fighting depression:
This book is dedicated to you. You are strong, brave, and resilient for facing this challenge head-on. Every step you take towards recovery, no matter how small, is a victory. May this book be a companion on your journey, offering hope, understanding, and tools to help you reclaim your life. You are not alone, and brighter days are ahead.

TABLE OF CONTENTS

CHAPTER 1

UNDERSTANDING DEPRESSION

Given that depression is more common in those who have a blood relative who also has the illness, depression is highly hereditary. Most likely, stress or life experiences can activate a genetic susceptibility that causes this. You are 1.5–3 times more likely to experience depression if you have a family member who does. Experiences in life frequently contribute to the start of sadness; yet, depression that manifests itself in the absence of these experiences is not unusual. Several life events, including the death of a parent or partner, becoming unemployed, getting hurt, or receiving a specific medical diagnosis, have been connected to depression. Depression can result from several what are known as cognitive biases and distortions that occur during various life experiences. An illustration of this might be someone. When someone is given a serious sickness diagnosis, they may not always believe that they are facing mortality. This type of thinking triggers an instinctive negative thought, which can then trigger the onset of depression.

Depression is a neurological condition. Many different brain pathways are not functioning well in the depression. Stress plays a role in the onset of depression, and that much is certain. Stress disrupts the brain's neurotransmitter systems, as we saw in the last section, which is why it frequently acts as a trigger for depression. Specifically, stress causes the hormone cortisol to be produced in excess. The amygdala's neurons are physically altered by this substance, which increases their sensitivity to negative input. The brain regions responsible for processing negative affect are hyperactive in depressed individuals, while the brain regions responsible for processing happy affect are underactive. This may cognitively result in a predisposition toward negativity in thought processes and an incapacity to shake off the pessimistic ideas linked to the start of depression.

The exact cause of depression, a very frequent and expensive condition that can hit at any time, is unknown. Although several psychiatric theories attempt to explain how depression develops, none of them is now complete. This could be the case because depression is not a single condition and can develop through a variety of pathways. Over the past 250 years, depression has afflicted humanity, and not much has changed. The ranking of depression as a cause of mortality in 1900 was the only notable shift. Heart disease is the only condition predicted to rank higher than depression by 2020 when depression was ranked 15th in the world. As for causes of mortality, depression is expected to rank second by then.

Ignoring ethnicities, nationalities, religions, and individual opinions, depression is a medical disorder and a global issue. It is regarded as one of the most prevalent ailments that affect every person. Individuals react differently to their biological and psychological states, and over time, this will cause more serious issues like illnesses, mental disorders, and even death.

1.1. What is Depression?

Bipolar disorder, dysthymia, and severe depression are the three primary forms of depression. Major depression, usually referred to as clinical depression, is a condition in which an individual has severe symptoms that make it difficult for them to function or enjoy life. The most prevalent kind of depression is this one. Long-term symptoms of dysthymia prevent a person from feeling well or functioning normally but do not render them disabled. This kind of depression can last for years, but because it is less severe and incapacitating, it is frequently dismissed. Mania, or extreme excitement, follows a depressive episode in bipolar illness patients' cycles. A person experiencing mania may feel incredibly joyful, strong, or agitated; occasionally, this is followed by a high-energy condition. When their symptoms are at their worst, people with bipolar disorder can be extremely productive, but they can also have terrible relationships or lose their jobs as a result.

Illnesses like depression are real. An estimated one in five adults (6.7%) suffer from depression each year, and one in six individuals (16.6%) will do so at some point in their lives. Though it can happen at any age, depression typically first manifests in late adolescence or early adulthood. Depression is more common in women than in males. According to certain research, one-third of women will go through a significant depressive episode at some point in their lives.

1.2. Causes of Depression

Early Life Events Childhood trauma or loss (like the death of a parent) can have a long-lasting effect, and adult and childhood experiences are frequently the root cause of depression. Depression can result from abuse at any age, whether it be sexual, emotional, or physical.

Events and Situations in Life The notion that depression can be brought on by "tough life circumstances" is not new. Indeed, sadness is regarded by many societies as one of the numerous "inevitable outcomes" of existence. Numerous events in life have the potential to negatively affect our mood, such as job loss, divorce, bereavement, money problems, or failing at   a   goal   we   set   out   to   achieve.

Biochemical   Elements   Moreover,   biochemical
abnormalities in the brain are believed to underlie
to contribute to depression. Depression is thought
to be caused by malfunctioning neurotransmitters
in the brain (e.g., not enough serotonin). This
explains why depression symptoms are frequently
relieved by medicine that modifies neurotransmitter
levels.

Genetic Contributions Certain individuals will have a
higher hereditary risk of depression because it can
run in families. It is important to note that having a
parent or close relative with depression does not
guarantee that an individual would also experience
depression. There is still a good chance that
personal circumstances and other factors will play a
significant role.

1.3. Signs and Symptoms of Depression
What is the Depression?

A persistent sense of melancholy or disinterest that
interferes   with   day-to-day   functioning   is   the

hallmark of major depressive disorder, a type of mood illness.

The following symptoms may be present:

- ❖ a sense of hopelessness or depression;
- ❖ a loss of interest in or enjoyment from previously enjoyed activities;
- ❖ changes in appetite or weight;
- ❖ difficulty sleeping or excessive sleep;
- ❖ exhaustion or energy loss;
- ❖ restlessness or a slowed-down sense of worthlessness or guilt;
- ❖ thoughts of death or suicide

It is imperative that you get expert care if you have five or more of these symptoms for a duration of two weeks or longer. Your quality of life can be greatly enhanced by an early diagnosis and course of   therapy. Furthermore, regardless of the existence of these symptoms, it a painful. It is a reality that parents' depression can have a major negative impact on their kids.

Depression symptoms can differ from person to person. This is because people differ greatly in terms of their personal characteristics, upbringing, and life experiences. But generally speaking, depression gets in the way of people's everyday lives and routines. One of the most prevalent signs of depression is excruciating mental suffering. The individual experiences this pain as a continual reminder of their inner emptiness.

1.4. Types of Depression

Depression is a phrase that can refer to a broad range of experiences rather than a single disease. When someone claims to be depressed, they typically mean what is referred to as severe depression or clinical depression in medicine. But there are several kinds of depression, and they can be brought on by a lot of different things. This segment of the website will examine the prevalent types of depression that are now recognized and treated. It is crucial to remember that not everyone experiences all of these symptoms at the same time, and they may not always indicate depression. We advise you to consult your family physician if you are not sure if this pertains to you. It is common for depression to coexist with other medical disorders. These can include Parkinson's disease, diabetes, cancer, HIV/AIDS, heart disease, and others. Additionally, it frequently coexists with other mental health issues. Anxiety is the most prevalent illness linked to depression. Depression and substance addiction disorders are frequently linked. There are situations where non-psychological factors might cause depression. Depression may arise as a result of a major life event, such as the death of a loved one, prolonged exposure to prejudice, or social isolation. An individual may be more vulnerable to a certain kind of depression depending on the underlying cause.

1.5 Laziness and Depression: A Complex Relationship

It's critical to realize that idleness is not a cause of depression, even though feelings of laziness and a lack of drive might be signs of the illness. This essay will investigate the complex connection between these two ideas, looking at the subtleties and providing more justifications for the demotivation that is frequently linked to depression.

Characterizing Depression and Laziness

- **Laziness**: The state of not wanting to do things or being motivated to do them. It may be arbitrary and impacted by individual tastes.
- **Depression**: A clinical mental health illness marked by enduring melancholy, diminished interest in or enjoyment of formerly enjoyed activities, and adjustments to sleep, food, and energy levels.

The Overlap: Why Depression Can Feel Like Laziness

<u>Primary Symptoms of Depression</u>:

Loss of Interest: One of the main signs of depression is a marked decline in interest or enjoyment in once-enjoyed activities. This can cause procrastination by making even simple chores seem daunting.

Fatigue and Low Energy: Depression can sap your energy, making even small chores seem extremely difficult. It's possible to mistake this lack of energy for lethargy.

Negative Thoughts: Feelings of worthlessness and negative self-talk are common companions of depression. People may become unmotivated to try as a result of this negativity since they may think they will fail in any case.

Anhedonia: One of the main signs of depression is the incapacity to feel joy. Activities that you used to like may now seem meaningless, which lowers motivation.

<u>For instance</u>: *Despite her enjoyment of trekking in the past, Sarah now finds the thought of putting on shoes tiresome. This lack of drive could be*

mistaken for laziness, but it could also be the result of *depression-related exhaustion.*

Depression's Fundamental Causes That Mirror Laziness

Biochemical Imbalances: Deregulation of some neurotransmitters, such as

Dopamine and serotonin affect energy levels, motivation, and mood.

Stressors in Life: Major life events such as a job loss, a change in relationships, or financial hardships can set off depression and make it harder to go through everyday life.

Medical illnesses: Some medical illnesses, such as thyroid issues or chronic fatigue syndrome, can have symptoms that mimic being lazy.

Overcoming the Label of Laziness

The Perils Associated with the Label of "Laziness":

Stigma: Calling someone a lazy person can stigmatize them and make them less likely to ask for assistance.

Self-Blame: People who are depressed may absorb the stigma associated with being lethargic, which can result in emotions of shame and guilt.

Importance of Accurate Diagnosis: Whether

depression or another problem is the root cause of a lack of motivation, a mental health specialist can accurately diagnose it.

Handsome Methods for Handling the Deficit in Motivation

Seeking Professional Assistance: A therapist can offer resources and encouragement to help manage depression and boost drive. Prescription drugs may also be given.

Dividing Up the Work: Big jobs might sometimes feel too much to handle. To boost motivation, break things down into smaller, more doable actions.

Put Progress First, Not Perfection:

Acknowledge and celebrate every little step forward you take. Positive behaviors are rewarded by this.

Creating a Support Network: Assemble a network of understanding and encouraging individuals around you to help you along the way.

Creating Healthful Habits: Give sleep, exercise, and a well-balanced diet a priority. These routines support increased vitality and general well-being.

In brief, although apathy and a lack of drive may be signs of depression, it's critical to identify the underlying causes. Through the implementation of healthy coping mechanisms and expert assistance, people can overcome obstacles and regain their motivation and overall well-being.

Additional Notes: The difficulties of attributing a lack of desire to laziness alone are the main topic of this research. True laziness, however, may also exist. For everyone, it's critical to strike a healthy balance between motivation and relaxation. Seek medical advice from a qualified practitioner in addition to this article. Please get help and direction from a mental health professional if you are experiencing low motivation.

1. 6 Marital Depression

Real or Imagined?

It's complicated to think that despair can follow marriage. It's crucial to understand the difference between correlation and causation, even though some people may feel a decrease in their happiness or mood following marriage. Below is a summary of the things to think about:

Is the Couple at Fault?

Previous Medical Conditions: Individuals who are prone to depression may be more inclined to wed someone who behaves dysfunctionally or has communication issues, which could exacerbate their sadness.

Irrational Expectations: When reality bites, romantic ideas about marriage might leave one feeling let down. It can be difficult to adjust to married life with all of its responsibilities, compromises, and in-law dynamics.

Life Transitions: Having children, purchasing a home, or taking on additional financial responsibilities are common life transitions that occur simultaneously with marriage. These pressures may aggravate a

A decrease in mood is not necessarily related to the union.

Communication Problems:

Ineffective communication, unsolved disputes, and a lack of emotional closeness can cause marital discontent and misery, which may hurt mental health.

Unmet Needs: Feelings of isolation, annoyance, and bitterness can arise in a married couple when emotional or physical needs aren't being satisfied, which can result in symptoms of depression. Difficulties versus Severe Depression:

Normal Adjustment Period: During the first few years of marriage, it's normal to face certain difficulties and make some adjustments. It's not always the case that this indicates clinical depression.

Severity and Length: Prolonged depressive sensations, a lack of interest in activities, and adjustments to sleep and eating patterns are the hallmarks of clinical depression. To make a diagnosis, these symptoms have to be present for a minimum of two weeks.

<u>Strengthening Your Marriage and Preventing Depression</u>:

Realistic Expectations: Before getting married, have an honest and open discussion about your expectations. Recognize that marriage is not always a picture-perfect romance and requires work.

Effective Communication: Work on your ability

to communicate clearly, learn how to assertively voice your wants, and engage in active listening. Preserve Individuality: Continue your interests, pastimes, and social life beyond marriage.

Put Quality Time First: Schedule frequent date evenings, group activities, and emotional closeness.

Preserve Good Habits: Give adequate rest, exercise, and a well-balanced diet top priority. These routines support resilience and general well-being.

Seek Professional Help: To address underlying issues, couples therapy or individual therapy may be helpful if communication is difficult or if depressed symptoms continue. Crucial Points to Remember:

• **Abuse**: Get assistance right away if you or your spouse are being verbally, physically, or emotionally abused in your marriage. It is not appropriate to attempt to resolve this issue on your own. You are deserving of respect and safety.

Put Your Attention on Answers: Rather than concentrating on the bad, find methods to strengthen your marriage and find answers.

In conclusion, depression is not caused by marriage per se. However certain difficulties and unfulfilled requirements in a marriage might lead to a deterioration in mood and well-being. Couples may overcome obstacles and create a loving and satisfying relationship by developing excellent communication skills, setting realistic expectations, and giving healthy coping methods priority. Whether you are depressed inside or outside of a marriage, getting expert therapy is essential.

Normal Adjustment Period: During the first few years of marriage, it's normal to face certain difficulties and make some adjustments. It's not always the case that this indicates clinical depression.

Intensity and Duration: Prolonged feelings of melancholy, a decline in interest in activities, and adjustments to sleep and eating are the hallmarks of clinical depression. To make a diagnosis, these symptoms have to be present for a minimum of two weeks.

1.7 A Complicated Web of Parenting Stress and Depression

Being a parent is undoubtedly hard, but it's also very rewarding. The never-ending expectations, insomniac evenings, and emotional ups and downs can wear parents out. Sometimes, this tension turns into depression, which has a serious negative effect on the health of both the parent and the child.

Recognizing the Connection:

Sleep Deprivation: The sleep rhythms of newborns and early children are disturbed, leaving parents exhausted all the time. Chronic sleep deprivation has been linked to depression symptoms such as exhaustion and difficulties focusing.

Social Isolation: Putting too much emphasis on child care may result in less social engagement with adults. The common symptoms of depression, such as feelings of isolation and loneliness, can be made worse by this lack of social interaction.

Financial Strain: Raising a child can come with a heavy financial cost. Concerned about One major source of stress that can exacerbate anxiety and sometimes even depression is money. **Identity Loss**: After having children, some parents find it difficult to cope with the change in who they are. Sadness and a lack of direction might result from someone feeling as though they've lost a piece of who they are.

Unrestricted Expectations: Idealized depictions of parenthood and societal pressures can lead to the development of unreasonable expectations. Constantly feeling inadequate can result in emotions of worthlessness and inadequacy, which are depressive symptoms.

Pre-existing Conditions: When faced with the extra stress of parenthood, parents who have a history of depression may be more susceptible to relapsing.

Parental Depression Symptoms:

Extended periods of melancholy, hopelessness, or irritation

A decrease in interest in or enjoyment of previously enjoyed activities, such as spending too much or too little time with your child; alterations in appetite or weight (weight gain or loss unrelated to dieting); trouble falling asleep; trouble focusing or making   decisions.

Suicidal or death-related thoughts frequently;

Energy loss or increasing weariness;

Feelings of guilt or worthlessness;

Safeguarding Your Health and Avoiding Depression:

Make self-care a priority. Even if it's only for a short while each day, set aside time for things you enjoy doing. To make time for self-care, ask for assistance with child care.

Seek Support: Discuss your difficulties with your spouse, family, and friends. Think about becoming a member of a parent support group.

Control Stress: To effectively control stress, engage in relaxation exercises like deep breathing or   meditation.

Preserve Good Habits: Eat a balanced diet, get regular exercise, and give sleep a priority. Your emotional and physical health is enhanced by these behaviors.

Have Realistic Expectations: Recognize that parenthood is difficult and messy, and let go of any exaggerated expectations. Appreciate minor successes and concentrate on development rather than perfection.

Seek Professional Assistance: Don't be afraid to get professional assistance if you're feeling depressed. A therapist can help you on your path to recovery by providing you with coping skills and encouragement.

Recall: You're not by yourself! A lot of parents feel overwhelmed and under stress. You can make parenting more enjoyable and rewarding for both you and your child by putting your health first, getting help when you need it, and learning how to handle stress.

CHAPTER 2

SEEKING HELP FOR DEPRESSION

2.1. Acknowledging the Need for Assistance

If you suffer from depression, as many people do, you might think you understand when you need assistance. For example, you might find it difficult to complete a task at work, or your spouse might be quite concerned that you are sleeping more than normal and that you are no longer doing things you used to like. You may already be aware of the detrimental impact depression's emotional and physical symptoms have on your life's quality. It can be exceedingly challenging to identify and accept the shortcomings and limits brought on by depression, though. Such acknowledgment is frequently an essential first step in obtaining therapy. When individuals with depression learn about their condition, they frequently dismiss the notion of receiving therapy. It can be difficult for them to recognize the possibility of feeling better and altering their perspective on the status quo if their melancholy mood is all they have ever known. It's easier said than done; for many, changing the notion of rehabilitation and returning to medicine is a big question. Usually, change and his perspective on things are challenging for them. It is essential to both contemplate and act upon it with great intensity. It will simply hold wounds and make an effort to heal, though. Acknowledging the need for treatment and acting upon it are crucial. Positive change requires a willingness to accept assistance. Admitting that you need help is difficult, but it is essential to your health. Although getting treatment might be a difficult task, doing so is a start in the right direction. You can find a wealth of information to aid you in your recovery process. Never hesitate to seek assistance. Recall that you are not fighting this battle alone. Some individuals wish to care about you.

Watch your recovery. Go for the assistance you require by taking the first step.

2.2. Talking to Experts in Mental Health

To find the best mental health practitioner for you, start by performing extensive research. Professional services are widely available, just as there are several types of mental diseases and the people who suffer from them. To significantly improve your chances of solving the issue, search for the best service for you; this may take some time and effort. Professionals having a specific concentration and technique for handling specific types of difficulties include clinical psychologists, counselors, and therapists; these are the most well-known.

Remember that the services are not all the same. For instance, a clinical psychologist will have a deeper understanding of the problems through psychological theories and will focus on treating a problem through methods like cognitive-behavior therapy; a counselor or therapist often works in general areas like helping to cope with life changes or developing coping strategies and emotional skills; this is often seen as a less intrusive service and is most often used by people who are not looking to resolve or understand a specific problem that is causing distress. A psychiatrist is primarily concerned with diagnosing an illness and prescribing and supervising a course of medication treatment.

2.3.   Resources   and   Support   Systems

It is hard to think that you will ever feel better when you are depressed. Even if you might think that your future is hopeless, it's crucial to understand that depression is a condition that can be treated. The correct kind of assistance can help with a lot of gloomy symptoms.

Having the support of friends and family might be crucial for depression recovery. You may feel worn out and powerless from depression, which will make you desire to isolate yourself from other people. Talking to someone you can trust can help you feel more appreciated, but isolating yourself can only make things worse. Conversely, the one you speak with need not be able to change you. All they have to do is listen well; that is, they should be able to hear you out without becoming sidetracked or passing judgment.

Support and self-help are important components of depression rehabilitation, but they shouldn't be your sole options for care. You might feel too worn out and depressed while you're under pressure to accomplish anything, hence getting by each day can seem like a daunting undertaking. For this reason, receiving expert depression treatment is essential. Depression can be extremely tough to conquer on its own, even though treatment might improve your mood and thought process. Proceed on your path to recovery; the sooner depression recedes, the less impact it will have on you.

CHAPTER 3

. COPING STRATEGIES FOR DEPRESSION

3.1 SELF CARE PRACTICES

Even if getting out of bed and doing something is tough when one is depressed, this is perhaps the best time to exercise self-care. When someone is depressed, they frequently cut self-care as the first item out of their daily schedule. Their depressive state sends the message that they are unworthy of attention and care. It is crucial to remember that we are susceptible to a variety of harmful coping strategies, including abusing drugs or alcohol, sleeping for excessively long periods, cutting ourselves off from friends, family, and activities, and overindulging in food. While withdrawing from others may provide momentary solace, interacting with others and participating in activities reenergizes and revitalizes us.

In the end, engaging in activities that lift our spirits, make us feel important, and give us a sense of success can help stop depression from setting in. Small, doable actions for yourself each day are the foundation of depression support and self-help. Begin by making an effort to comprehend that the sole sign of depression that hinders a person's capacity to assist themselves, which further fuels hopelessness, is hopelessness. It is a vicious cycle that can be broken by making tiny progress toward modest objectives, which in turn fosters optimism and self-efficacy. You can and will overcome depression by using the tools in this guide and putting them into practice daily. Attempting to include some of the following self-care practices is the first step into your existence. Start small and work your way up to greater activities. Avoid taking on too much at once because feeling depressed is often a result of overworking yourself and failing. To increase the likelihood of success, implement these methods gradually. Recall that while changing one's life is difficult, it is necessary to overcome depression. Big progress with little steps.

3.2. Healthy Lifestyle Habits

Numerous details regarding the management of depression symptoms and the creation of a healthy and productive lifestyle may be found in the literature study. It is recommended to engage in regular physical activity, consume a diet high in omega-3 fatty acids, get lots of sleep, etc. Depression can be effectively treated by incorporating these practices into one's everyday routine.

3.2.1. Frequent Exercise

Engaging in consistent physical activity is crucial for individuals with mild to moderate depression symptoms, and it can serve as a supplement for those suffering from severe depression. The research on depression frequently indicates that physical activity can help lessen depressive symptoms. It implies that engaging in 150 minutes a week of moderate-intensity exercise enhances mood and sleep quality. Research on sad adults with ages ranging from Research 50 and 77 demonstrated that a 4-month physical exercise regimen reduced depressive symptoms. Finding things that one enjoys doing is essential for motivation. Exercise can be done in a variety of ways, both by yourself and with others. Walking in a park and engaging in physical activity can be combined with relaxing techniques to create an outdoor exercise program. A few minutes of vigorous aerobic exercise first thing in the morning will help you feel more in control and happier all day. Compared to non-aerobic exercise, aerobic exercise is seen to be a more useful strategy for treating depression. The first study to compare exercise and medication was done by Blumenthal et al., and they discovered that an exercise regimen was just as effective as taking anti-depressants. The exercise group experienced fewer relapses than the medication-taking patients, despite the latter group's greater rates of remission. Finally, achieving goals and witnessing improvements in one's physical fitness can greatly contribute to the development of self-esteem through exercise.

3.2.2. Consumption

According to published research, those who experience depressive symptoms are more prone to eat a diet poor in nutrients. A diet heavy in fat and fast food consumption raises the risk of depression. Dietary habits and depression risk were also highlighted in the research. A diet high in red meat, desserts, sweets, soft drinks, fried food, processed food, refined cereals, and an unhealthy eating pattern were all linked to an elevated risk of depression. A balanced diet that emphasizes fruits, vegetables, seafood, and whole grains has been linked to a lower incidence of depression. 12,059 participants in Spanish observational research who had the highest adherence to Depression risk were shown to be 30% lower in those following a Mediterranean diet. This gave rise to theories that diet modifications can lessen depressive symptoms. A 10-day food intervention was evaluated to see if it affected the symptoms of severe depression in both male and female convicts in a New Zealand trial. During the course of those ten days, it was discovered that the group fed processed food had an increased risk of depression of 50–100% (depending on the individual) compared to the group fed high-quality whole food, which had a decreased risk of depression of 20–30% (depending on the individual). Lastly, because diet modification intervention is feasible, nutrition affects depression, and making dietary changes can help people feel better physically as well as less depressed.

3.3. Cognitive Behavioral Techniques

This method strongly adheres to the idea that a guy should be taught how to fish rather than being handed one. Through this type of therapy, the client can identify and correct cognitive errors that may be leading to poor behavior and, ultimately, depression. All-or-nothing thinking, for instance, is a common distortion observed in depressed clients. It goes something like this: "I have either done this job perfectly, or I am a total failure." The client can break out from this habit with the therapist's assistance, which will enable them to approach the work with greater flexibility and, ultimately, produce better results.

The cognitive-behavioral task of arranging tasks is another example of boosting happiness or a feeling of accomplishment. People who are depressed often retreat from social interactions, and even a small setback might reinforce their sense that they are completely incapable of doing anything. Through the establishment of modest and practically attainable objectives, like paying a visit to a friend or finishing a minor household chore, the client can enhance their self-confidence and lessen the consequences of setbacks. This is frequently used in conjunction with graded task assignments when a difficult activity is broken down into smaller, more manageable steps by the therapist and client. The client can start applying what they've learned to other projects after they've seen firsthand how addressing work in this way reduces stress and produces better results.

3.4. Mindfulness and Meditation

While there are many different ways to meditate, they all aim to quiet the mind's racing thoughts. There are several advantages, including improved focus, a stronger capacity to manage stress, heightened immunity, elevated self-awareness, and an all-around sense of well-being. The brain ages more slowly when it is not under stress because a less stressed mind functions more efficiently. Enter the "space between your thoughts," through meditation, can be beneficial to both the mind and the body. Four components are similar to most forms of meditation: a calm environment, a particular, comfortable posture, concentrated concentration, and an open mindset. A mental exercise called mindfulness can help one become more aware of the present moment. It entails deliberately opening up, engaging in, and being responsive to your present-moment experience. It is a great remedy for the tendency to sleepwalk through life that depression is known to cause. A common misconception among those who experience it is that it entails trying to "think positive thoughts" or adopting an "I'm OK, you're OK" mindset. This mindset will lessen self-awareness, self-acceptance, and self-compassion—the same qualities required to cleanse the mind of suffering. You are not aiming to reach a particular level of relaxation or run away from any uncomfortable or upsetting thoughts or emotions while you are aware. As an alternative, you learn to accept and empathize with the ideas and feelings by learning to be with them. Being mindful entails accepting one's thoughts and emotions for what they are, developing awareness of them, and developing a clearer understanding of them. Being mindful

Being more conscious is all that meditation does without. When meditation is effective, conscious awareness follows naturally. Being mindful is paying attention and being present consciously and purposefully. Acting carelessly, uninformed, and aimlessly is the opposite of this. The awareness required to be mindful is developed by meditation.

CHAPTER 4
TREATMENT OPTIONS FOR DEPRESSION

Important Information

Disclaimer:

This information is not intended to be used as medical advice; rather, it is for educational purposes only. Please get in touch with a licensed mental health professional for assistance if you are experiencing depression.

4.1. Comprehending Depression Medication

Even though depression typically has a detrimental impact on one's feelings, thoughts, and behavior, there are thankfully efficient remedies, including medicine. This guide will examine the many kinds of depression drugs, their modes of action, adverse effects, and resources for additional support. How Can Depression Be Helped by Medication? Serotonin and norepinephrine imbalances in particular have been related to depression. To elevate mood and reduce symptoms, medications control these substances. Different Depression Drug Types There are numerous drug classifications in use for depression, each has a unique side effect profile and mode of action. Below is a summary of the most prevalent ones:

SSRIs, or selective serotonin reuptake inhibitors: These are the antidepressants that are most frequently given. SSRIs function by preventing serotonin from being reabsorbed in the brain.

increasing serotonin availability. Sertraline (Zoloft), citalopram (Celexa), fluoxetine (Prozac), escitalopram (Lexapro), and paroxetine (Paxil) are a few examples. In addition to acting similarly to SSRIs, serotonin-norepinephrine reuptake inhibitors (SNRIs) also alter norepinephrine levels in the brain. Venlafaxine (Effexor) and duloxetine (Cymbalta) are two examples.

Tricyclic Antidepressants (TCAs): SSRIs and SNRIs are more likely to have fewer adverse effects than TCAs, an older family of antidepressants that is no longer as widely prescribed. They may, however, be helpful for certain individuals, especially those who have severe depression or have not responded to previous treatments. Amitriptyline (Elavil), imipramine (Tofranil), and nortriptyline (Pamelor) are a few examples.

Monoamine oxidase inhibitors (MAOIs): Because of possible conflicts with specific foods and drugs, MAOIs are a very effective class of antidepressants that are not administered as frequently. They function by preventing the breakdown of monoamines, including dopamine, serotonin, and norepinephrine. Phenelzine (Nardil) and tranylcypromine (Parnate) are two examples.

Unconventional Antidepressants: These drugs don't readily fit into another group. While some employ special methods, others blend the impacts of several kinds. Trazodone (Desyrel), bupropion (Wellbutrin), and mirtazapine (Remeron) are a few examples.

Selecting the Appropriate Drug
The optimal kind of medicine for you will depend on several things, such as your medical history, response to prior therapies, and symptoms. You will collaborate with a mental health expert, like a therapist or psychiatrist, to choose the right drug and dose.

Taking Medication for Depression

The following are important things to keep in mind when using depression medication:

Working can take some time: If you don't feel better right away, don't give up. It usually takes a few weeks for antidepressants to have full effect.

Avoid stopping your medicine suddenly: Withdrawal symptoms may occur if antidepressants are stopped abruptly. Before altering your prescription schedule, always get your doctor's approval.

Adverse consequences: Side effects are possible with all drugs. Typical adverse reactions to antidepressants include nausea, dry mouth, erectile dysfunction, and insomnia. These usually get better with time. Notify your physician of any persistent or troublesome side effects.

Frequent arrivals: Make routine check-ups with your physician so they can assess your condition and, if needed, modify your prescription. Extra Things to Think About Although medicine might be a potent tool for treating depression, which works best when paired with other therapies like counseling in addition to addressing underlying problems that might be causing your sadness, therapy can help you learn coping skills and enhance your general well-being.

4.2. Psychotherapy Approaches

Everyone plays a role in their own life, making life a play. A person's experience of not the greatest part of an act is what gives rise to feelings of sadness and depression. Just like actors would want advice and support to enhance the part they play, sad people would also require it. Psychotherapy provides depressed people with guidance and suggestions on how to overcome their depression, which is just what they would need.

Psychotherapy comes in a variety of forms for those who suffer from depression. Interpersonal, psychodynamic, and cognitive-behavioral therapies are among the psychotherapy clusters. Cognitive-behavioral therapy has been the treatment with the greatest research on treating depression. It is the outcome of behavioral psychology and cognitive therapy combined. Mental While behavioral therapy teaches patients how to use specific skills in the identification and modification of behaviors, cognitive therapy teaches patients how to think clearly and examine their thoughts. Cognitive behavior therapists work to alter unfavorable thought processes that are assumed to exacerbate depression in their patients. Relapse prevention may be significantly aided by the genetic influence on cognitive change, according to a recent investigation. In addition to teaching patients how to be their therapists, the goal of therapy is to reduce current symptoms and provide long-lasting benefits. When it comes to treating mild depression, cognitive therapy is just as effective as antidepressant drugs. Its effects last longer, with considerably reduced rates of recurrence over the next six to twelve months. The lowest dropout rate is seen with this therapy rate about alternative treatment modalities. Those who are highly susceptible to depression can also benefit from the preventive application of the cognitive treatment package. Due to its active structure and the behavioral focus of atypical depression, behavioral therapy may be a beneficial addition to cognitive treatment for depression, despite the latter's greater testing. This therapy is primarily practical in nature and focuses on teaching certain skills. Therapy based on cognitive behavior is

When it comes to educating the client and helping them understand and apply what they have learned, homework in between sessions is highly valued, as is the patient's development of long-lasting and trans-situational coping mechanisms.

4.3. Complementary and Alternative Medicine

Alternative therapies, many of which apply to depression, seek to allay anxiety and resolve problems. Certain activities help people feel less depressed and more in control of their lives by counteracting the symptoms of depression. For instance, one of the most typical signs of depression is feeling powerless. It has been suggested that learning to drum can help people feel more empowered and less depressed. Recently, a technique for treating depression that involved an aerobic workout form developed by Cooper Institute colleagues was successful.

Exercise that is aerobic in nature is one that, if continued for a It has been demonstrated to improve mood for at least 30 minutes. Finding the motivation to begin and finish the exercise is the hardest part of dealing with depression. The National Institute of Mental Health experimented to create an exercise program that is simple to begin and maintain for those with poor motivation. This led to the development of hatha yoga as a depression treatment method. The participants were split into two groups: one practiced yoga, while the other engaged in walking, a well-known aerobic activity. At one, three, and six-month intervals, the anxiety and depressed mood of both groups were compared. At each interval, the walking group's anxiety and despair decreased less than those of the yoga group. A successful strategy for lessening the effects of depression would be to look for other pursuits that produce similar outcomes. Choosing to employ alternative therapies should be carefully considered.

Taking into account the extent of the depression and the current conventional treatments. Safe and encouraging surroundings can be used to deliver a variety of alternative therapies. This may apply to music or group art classes. These can be uplifting encounters that offer a channel for feelings that would otherwise be incomprehensible. When it comes to minor forms of melancholy, these kinds of activities are usually the safest alternative therapies. However, substituting standard depression treatments with alternative ones that are taken internally or topically has a higher risk. Herbal supplements and drug cessation are two examples of these, as are alternative therapies that might only be accessible in particular regions or nations. Seeking the advice of a physician is highly recommended.

The doctor can assist create a well-informed plan of action and advice on whether an alternative therapy will interfere with existing treatments.

4.4. Inpatient and Hospital Programs

Depression Hospitalization and Inpatient Programs

When receiving extensive treatment for depression, an individual stays at a hospital or treatment center for the whole course of their program. This is known as inpatient care. For those with severe depression who:

Cannot take care of themselves due to severe symptoms (eating, hygiene);

Have not responded effectively to outpatient treatment;

Pose a risk to themselves or others (suicidal ideas or plans);

Advantages of inpatient care

Constant oversight and assistance: offers a secure setting under constant observation to reduce the danger of suicide and meet necessities.

Concentrate on stabilization: This enables rapid improvements in mood and functioning through intense therapy and drug changes.

Elimination of stressors: Reduces everyday strains that exacerbate depression.

Program types for inpatients:

Voluntary admission: When a patient decides to check into a hospital.

Involuntary admission: To avoid injury in extreme circumstances, a physician or mental health specialist may advise involuntary hospitalization. Local laws differ.

Anticipations for an inpatient program:

Evaluation: Physicians evaluate patients' symptoms, and medical histories, and create a plan of care.

Individual therapy: Consistent appointments to work on coping mechanisms and address ideas and feelings.

Group therapy: Assists with social skill development and offers peer support.

Medication management: To control symptoms, doctors may start or modify medication. Options for care outside of hospitalization include

Outpatient therapy: Consistent visits with a while residing in one's own house.

Programs for partial hospitalization (PHPs): intense therapy during the day, with evenings and nights spent at home. Locating an inpatient program: Speak with your physician or a mental health specialist.

Mental health hotlines and websites can offer information and support.

Look for internet listings of mental health facilities in your area that take your insurance.

Recall: *You're not by yourself. Inpatient care can*

be a crucial step on the road to recovery for those with depression, which is a treatable disorder.

CHAPTER 5

MANAGING DEPRESSION IN DAILY LIFE

5.1. Building a Supportive Routine

What is a Supportive Routine?

Establishing a dependable and regimented daily schedule might be an effective strategy for overcoming depression. This is about creating good habits that provide you stability and a sense of achievement, not strict micromanagement.

Advantages of a Helpful Schedule:

Diminishes Choice Fatigue: Reduces the mental strain of having to decide what to do next every day, which frees up energy to manage depressive symptoms.

Encourages Consistency: Mood enhancement and general well-being are enhanced by regular sleep, eating, and exercise regimens.

Enhances Self-Esteem: Finishing activities and maintaining a schedule give one a sense of self-worth and control.

Enhances Sleep: Regular sleep routines aid in the regulation of sleep patterns, which has a profound effect on mood.

Creating a Routine:

1. **Begin Little**: Avoid taking on too much. Start with one or two small, doable activities, such as establishing a regular time for waking up.

2. **Remain Basic**: Give adequate rest, wholesome food, and frequent exercise a priority. Increases in physical exercise, even modest ones, can lift your spirits.

3. **Plan Pleasurable Activities**: Allocate time for hobbies, social engagement, or enjoyable relaxation methods.

4. **Remain Adaptable**: Life occurs! As much as possible, strive for consistency, but be willing to make modifications.

5. **Monitor Your Development**: Keep track of your mood and routine compliance with a journal or app. Enjoy your victories and make necessary adjustments.

Recall that it takes time and practice to establish a helpful routine. Have patience with yourself, and don't be scared to ask for expert advice if you need more direction. Here are a few more pointers:

Include close relatives: Tell your loved ones

about your regimen and solicit their assistance. **Treat yourself**: Recognize your efforts with modest incentives for maintaining your schedule. **Commence your day victorious**: Start the day with a straightforward activity completed to gain momentum and a positive outlook. You can regain control over your day and more skillfully handle the symptoms of depression by establishing a beneficial routine.

5.2. Cultivating Connections

Depression can have a lasting effect on your relationships' health as well as your well-being. Relationships with loved ones may be strained by the social disengagement, poor energy, and negativity that come with depression. Nonetheless, solid connections that provide support, motivation, and a feeling of community are essential for rehabilitation.

Here are some tips for maintaining relationships while dealing with depression: Recognizing Depression's Effects

Difficulties in Communicating: Depression can make it difficult to communicate honestly and openly. You could become withdrawn from discussions or find it difficult to communicate your needs and emotions.

Emotional Withdrawal: Neglecting relationships with loved ones can result from a wish to withdraw emotionally.

Enhanced Irritability: Depression can exacerbate your irritability and make you more easily agitated, which can affect how you interact with other people.

Loss of Interest: Past Favorite Activities with Family members may become less appealing, causing a rift.

Techniques for Developing Partnerships

Honest and Open Communication: Discuss your depression with your loved ones. Describe the difficulties you're having and how they could influence your actions.

Have Reasonable Expectations: Advise them that you might require more time and assistance. Remind them that you're devoted to getting healthier even though rehabilitation takes time.

Make active listening a habit: Give your loved

ones your full attention when they express concern, and acknowledge their emotions.

Emphasize Quality Time: Even if it's just a brief but deep chat, making time for loved ones should be your priority. Quantity is important, but so is quality.

Control Expectations: Don't count on flawless relationships. Depression can lead to conflict, but difficulties can be overcome with effort and open communication. Tips for Effective Communication

Make "I" Declarations: Express how your depression affects you, rather than placing blame on others (e.g., "I feel withdrawn because of my depression, but I value our connection").

Concentrate on Particular Needs: Make it clear what kind of assistance you require. Do you need someone to go with you to appointments, provide distractions, or listen to you?

Practice self- and other-compassion: Clear communication requires reciprocity. Allow your family members some time to comprehend sadness and modify their expectations.

Keeping   Healthy   Distinctions

It's Acceptable to Deny: Energy can be depleted by depression. If you're not up for an invitation, don't be scared to turn it down.

Express Your Needs: Tell those you care about when you need time to yourself or assistance to go to social events.

• **Establish Boundaries with Negativity**: Restrict your interactions with people who are unhelpful or judgmental. Be in the company of understanding and encouraging individuals. Getting Help for the People You Love

• **Educate Them**: Give your loved ones some reading material on depression. They can learn about the illness and how to support others by using resources like support groups or mental health websites.

Promote Therapy: Take into account going to family or couple's therapy sessions jointly. A therapist can help with conflict resolution, communication guidance, and strengthening support networks.

Support Groups: Family support groups for those with depression can facilitate relationships between loved ones and others going through comparable struggles.

Self-Care: The Cornerstone of Sturdy Partnerships Keeping yourself well is crucial to preserving happy relationships. You have greater energy when your health is your top priority and the ability to emotionally bond with people.

Adhere to a Healthy Routine: Sleep, eating a balanced diet, and exercising regularly are essential for mood enhancement and depression management.

Therapy: Therapy can help you develop coping mechanisms, deal with unfavorable thought habits, and strengthen your emotional fortitude. Medication: Antidepressant medications, when recommended by a physician, can greatly enhance your mood and general state of health. **Mindfulness Techniques**: Deep breathing techniques, yoga, and meditation can help reduce stress and enhance emotional control. Recall that maintaining healthy connections while treating depression calls for work on the part of you and your loved ones. Practice self- and other-compassion, place a high value on honest communication, and get help from professionals when necessary. Good relationships provide love, support, and a feeling of community during trying times, making them an effective aid for rehabilitation.

5.3. Handling the Delicate Balance Between Work and Personal Life:

Depression Work and Personal Life: The pernicious effects of depression can affect all aspects of your life, not just your mood. your life—including your career and interpersonal connections When combating depression, finding a good balance between these two areas becomes even more important. Here are some tips for executing this delicate dance:

Recognizing the Obstacles:

Decreased Energy: Depression can drain your energy, making it hard to meet obligations at work and participate in leisure activities more

Difficulties Focusing: It might be difficult to stay focused on tasks, which can affect how well you perform at work and how much you enjoy your hobbies.

Negative Self-Talk: Depression-related inner critics can undermine interpersonal connections and create feelings of inadequacy at work.

Loss of Interest: Past passions may become less appealing, leaving you feeling separation from your personal life and seclusion.

Work-Life Intrusion: Bringing work stress home or continuously checking emails can cause you to lose sleep and become less relaxed. Techniques for a Better Equilibrium:

Make self-care a priority. Getting enough sleep, eating well, and exercising are the cornerstones of controlling depression and enhancing your capacity to handle obligations from both your personal and professional life.

Set Boundaries: Clearly define the lines separating your personal and professional lives. After work hours, disconnect from job-related calls and emails.

Communicate with Your Employer: Discuss your depression with your supervisor, if at all feasible. To relieve some of the strain, look at solutions like lower workloads or flexible work schedules.

Time Management Skills: Acquire efficient time management skills to prioritize professional responsibilities and make time for personal pursuits you find satisfying.

Assign and Request Help: Don't be embarrassed to assign chores to coworkers or request assistance. The weight can be lessened by sharing it.

Plan Your Activities: Set out time on your calendar for things you enjoy doing, including hanging out with friends and family, taking up a new hobby, or just unwinding.

Develop Your Ability to Say No: Avoid taking on too many obligations outside of work. Refusing invites is acceptable if you require personal time.

<u>Work-Life Harmony and Treatment of Depression</u>:

Therapy: You can develop resilience, enhance communication skills, and manage negative thought patterns with the help of cognitive-behavioral therapy (CBT).

Medication: If prescribed by a physician, antidepressants can greatly elevate your mood and energy levels, facilitating the management of both personal and professional obligations.

Support Groups: Making connections with people who are cognizant of the difficulties associated with depression can yield invaluable assistance and motivation.

Strengthening Interpersonal Connections: **Honest Communication**: Discuss your depression with your loved ones. Describe the difficulties you're having and how they could influence your actions.

Emphasize Quality Time: Even if it's just a brief but deep chat, making time for loved ones should be your priority. Quantity is important, but so is quality.

Have Reasonable Expectations: Advise them that you might require additional time and assistance. Remind them that you're devoted to getting healthier even though rehabilitation takes time.

Engage in Active Listening: Pay close attention to what loved ones are saying and acknowledge their emotions.

Recall that striking a healthy work-life balance is a journey, not a destination. extend further There will be days when your personal life needs to change due to increased job responsibilities. Treat yourself well, and don't be embarrassed to seek assistance when you need it. Despite the difficulties of depression, you can design a more balanced and meaningful life by putting your health first, establishing healthy boundaries, and getting help from a professional when necessary. Never forget that you are not traveling alone.

5.4.   Making   sensible   objectives

It's even more crucial to create reasonable goals when battling depression. Here's how to modify the procedure to get around the difficulties that depression brings:

Recognize Your Present Situation: **Accurately state what your present constraints are**. Make sure your goals are not too high to avoid setting yourself up for failure because depression can sap ambition and energy. **Pay Attention to Baby, Doable Steps**: Begin with little, manageable initiatives rather than striving for a total lifestyle makeover.

This may be taking a shower after getting out of bed, going for a fifteen-minute walk, or doing one task each day.

Make Self-Care Your Top Priority: Your first objective may just be to create wholesome sleep, eating, and exercise routines. **Managing your health is the first step** toward developing resilience in your despondency.

Prioritize Progress Over Perfection: Honor **even the tiniest successes**. Important victories can include doing a chore you've been putting off, going to a therapy session, or even just getting dressed.

Break Down Bigger Objectives: Divide long-term objectives into weekly or monthly benchmarks, such as going back to work or taking up a new pastime.

A goal of going back to work might, for instance, include benchmarks such as updating your résumé, reaching out to a few potential employers, or participating in a class on job interview techniques.

Be Kind and Adaptable to Yourself: Unpredictable relapses are possible with depression. Accept that healing is a slow process and don't be hard on yourself if you experience setbacks or need to modify your goals. Examples of Practical Depression Goals

Handle with care: Go to bed by 11 p.m. and get up by 8 a.m. every day. Consume two healthful snacks and three well-balanced meals per day. Three times a week, go for a 20-minute stroll.

Therapy: Show up for all of your arranged sessions. Finish any exercises or assignments that your therapist has given you.

Social Interaction: Make one weekly phone call to a friend or relative. Once a month, take part in a virtual support group.

Level of Activity: Spend five minutes every morning doing deep breathing exercises. Twice a week, do a 10-minute yoga practice.

Extra Advice: Consult Your Therapist: Talk to your therapist about your objectives. They can support you while you strive for your objectives and assist you in setting reasonable ones.

Monitor Your Progress: Keep note of your progress using a journal or an app toward your objectives. Observing your successes can inspire you.

Reward Yourself: Select modest prizes for reaching your objectives. This keeps you motivated and reinforces good conduct. Recall that one of the most effective strategies for treating depression is to set reasonable goals. Through self-compassion, self-care as a top priority, and an emphasis on tiny victories, you may progressively gain ground and pave the way for a better tomorrow.

6. Overcoming Challenges in Depression

Depression is a long-lasting shadow that affects relationships, energy, motivation, and mood. It can be debilitating, as though you're caught in a never-ending circle of pessimism and despair. The good news is that depression is a disorder that can be treated. You can recover your life and conquer the obstacles it brings if you have the correct resources and assistance.

You'll get tools and techniques from this guide to help you on your journey to recovery.

We'll investigate:

Recognizing Depression: Acquire knowledge of the signs, origins, and varieties of depression.

Establishing a Supportive Routine: Learn how discipline and well-being practices can help you take charge of your depression management.

Creating Coping Mechanisms: Arm yourself with strategies for handling stress, unpleasant feelings, and thoughts.

Taking Care of Relationships: Discover how to keep wholesome bonds with those you care about while fighting depression.

Balancing Work and Personal Life: Learn how

to take care of your mental health while managing the responsibilities of your job.

Setting Realistic Goals: Learn how to create attainable objectives that advance development and boost self-confidence.

Obtaining Professional Assistance: Discover the various forms of therapy available and how to locate a licensed mental health practitioner. Recall that you are not fighting this battle alone. Millions of people suffer from depression, and countless more have overcome their illness. This guide is intended to provide you with the necessary skills, support, and encouragement to help you overcome the obstacles of depression and take back your life.

6.1. Dealing with Stigma and Misunderstanding

Depression is a long-lasting shadow that affects relationships, energy, motivation, and mood. It can be debilitating, as though you're caught in a never-ending circle of pessimism and despair. The good news is that depression is a disorder that can be treated. You can recover your life and conquer the obstacles it brings if you have the correct resources and assistance.

You'll get tools and techniques from this guide to help you on your journey to recovery. We'll investigate:

Recognizing Depression: Acquire knowledge of the signs, origins, and varieties of depression.

Establishing a Supportive Routine: Learn how discipline and well-being practices can help you take charge of your depression management.

Creating Coping Mechanisms: Arm yourself with strategies for handling stress, unpleasant feelings, and thoughts.

Taking Care of Relationships: Discover how to keep wholesome bonds with those you care about while fighting depression.

Balancing Work and Personal Life: Learn how to take care of your mental health while managing the responsibilities of your job.

Setting Realistic Goals: Learn how to create attainable objectives that advance development and boost self-confidence.

Obtaining Professional Assistance: Discover the various forms of therapy available and how to locate a licensed mental health practitioner. Recall that you are not fighting this battle alone. Millions of people suffer from depression, and countless more have overcome their illness. This guide is intended to provide you with the necessary skills, support, and encouragement to help you overcome the obstacles of depression and take back your life.

6.2. Dealing with Slip-ups and Failures

Managing Depression Relapses and Setbacks: Keeping Up Your Pace

Recovery from depression is rarely a straight-line path. Even with medical intervention and effective coping strategies in place, you may have setbacks or relapses. Though they can be depressing, it's crucial to keep in mind that they are a typical stage of the procedure. Let's look at some helpful methods for dealing with setbacks and relapses: Gratitude Recurrences versus Delays: **Relapses**: These are notable episodes of depression that recur and can extend for several days, weeks, or even months. They frequently entail reverting to the behavioral habits you were trying to alter, including ignoring your own needs or isolating yourself from others. **Setbacks**: These are brief, perhaps multi-day drops in motivation or attitude. They usually don't make a big difference in your total progress.

Recognizing Early Warning Signs: By being aware of your warning indicators, you can take action before a possible setback or relapse takes hold. The following are typical warning signs to look out for:

Modifications in Sleep or Appetite: Sleep disturbances, excessive sleeping, or adjustments in eating patterns may be the first indications of a mood change.

Increasing Social Isolation: Refusing to interact with loved ones or participate in social events can be a red flag.

Negative Self-Talk: A discernible rise in self-deprecating ideas about oneself or the future may indicate an impending setback.

Loss of Interest: A decline in mood may be indicated by a loss of interest in once-enjoyed activities.

Decreased Energy: Excessive fatigue or a lack of drive may be red flags.

Techniques for Handling Setbacks and Relapses:

Speak with Your Support System: Share your feelings with friends, family, and your therapist. Their encouragement and support might be quite helpful.

Examine Your Course of Treatment: Talk to your therapist about any changes in your symptoms. They may need to change the way you take your medicine or receive therapy.

Emphasize self-care: Give regular exercise, a balanced diet, and restful sleep a top priority. These routines offer a basis for managing emotional difficulties.

Work on Your Relaxation Skills: Progressive muscle relaxation, mindfulness meditation, and deep breathing techniques can all aid in stress management and mood enhancement.

Make Use of Your Coping Strategies: Use the coping mechanisms you have acquired in treatment to properly handle your negative thoughts and feelings.

Try to keep things as regular as you can:

Maintaining your daily schedule as much as you can, despite modifications, can provide you with a sense of stability in the face of adversity.

Be Kind to Yourself: If you have a setback, don't punish yourself. Recognize the difficulties and return your attention to your healing process.

<u>Relapse Prevention in the Future</u>:

Early Intervention: Take quick action in response to early warning indicators to stop a small setback from getting worse.

Recognize Stressors: Determine stressful life situations that could set off depressive episodes and devise coping mechanisms for them.

Sustain Treatment: Avoid stopping medicine or therapy too soon. For depression to be managed over the long term, consistent treatment is essential.

Keep Developing Resilience: To improve your emotional health, engage in self-care, coping mechanisms, and constructive self-talk routines.

Create a Relapse Prevention Plan: Together with your therapist, come up with a customized plan that identifies triggers, warning indicators, and coping mechanisms for potential problems down the   road.

Recall that setbacks and relapses do not indicate failure; rather, obstacles in the path of healing. You can overcome these obstacles and continue moving in the direction of a happier and healthier life if you have the correct support system, employ practical techniques, and make time for yourself. You may overcome the difficulties associated with depression and restore your mental health by being knowledgeable, taking initiative, and getting help when you need it.

6.3. Handling Conditions That Co-occur

Handling Co-Occurring Disorders: A Useful Manual

Many people deal with two or more mental health conditions at the same time, rather than just one. We refer to these as co-occurring conditions. Depression and anxiety disorders, eating disorders and mood disorders, substance use disorders, and post-traumatic stress disorder (PTSD) are common combinations.

Co-occurring condition challenges:

Because symptoms from one ailment might exacerbate those from the other, co-occurring conditions can be more difficult to treat than single conditions. Depression, for instance, can exacerbate appetites for substances, while substance abuse can exacerbate feelings of anxiety.

The course of treatment for one illness may conflict with that for another. Reluctance to seek treatment can result from feeling overwhelmed by several illnesses. Successful Techniques for Handling Co-occurring Circumstances:

1. **Integrated Treatment:** For co-occurring illnesses, this is the most successful strategy. To treat every ailment at once, a group of experts must collaborate. A psychiatrist, therapist, counselor, and primary care physician could be on this team.

Take Action: Look for a therapist or treatment facility with experience providing integrated care for co-occurring conditions.

2. **Make self-care a priority:**

Maintaining good sleep, eating a balanced diet, and exercising regularly are essential for handling the mental and physical strain of co-occurring diseases.

Take Action: Create a daily schedule that includes these healthful practices and try your best to follow it.

3. **Communication Is Essential**:

It's crucial to be completely honest and open with your treatment team about all of your experiences and symptoms.

Take Action: Ask questions if you have any and be open about your difficulties when nothing is clear. Your staff will be better able to customize care the more they comprehend your particular circumstance.

4. **Deal with the Root Causes**: Substance abuse disorders and poor coping strategies frequently arise as a means of managing the underlying emotional distress associated with another illness, such as PTSD or depression. Taking care of the underlying cause is essential for long-term healing.

Take Action: Investigate the underlying problems

causing your co-occurring conditions by working with your therapist.

5. **Develop Effective Coping Skills**: You may handle triggers and deal with obstacles in a healthy way by learning healthy coping mechanisms including mindfulness exercises, relaxation techniques, and stress management tactics.

Take Action: Discuss learning and using evidence-based coping techniques with your therapist.

6. **Establish a Robust Support Network**: Assemble a network of understanding and encouraging friends, relatives, or support groups.

Take Action: Establish connections with others who are aware of co-occurring conditions and who can provide support and encouragement.

7. **Have Self-Compassion and Be** Patient: Healing is a process, not a finish line. There are going to be obstacles in the path. Be kind, acknowledge your accomplishments, and don't hesitate to ask for more help when you need it.

Take Action: Show yourself compassion and give yourself credit for managing these challenging conditions.

By being proactive, getting support from a

professional, and putting these useful methods into practice, you may manage co-occurring disorders well and pave the way for a happier, healthier life.

CHAPTER 7

THRIVING BEYOND DEPRESSION

Overcoming Depression: Regaining Your Life and Health

Depression can have a lasting effect on your energy, mood, and general sense of well-being. The good news is that depression is a disorder that can be treated. You may overcome depression and make a full recovery with the correct resources and assistance. This book will provide you with the tools and techniques you need to go beyond simply existing and experience true success in life. Changing the Way You See Things:

You Are Not Defined by Depression: Your diagnosis does not define you. Depression need not characterize who you are as a person, even though it could be a part of your path.

Put Growth First: Recovering offers a chance to advance personally. You can strengthen your resilience, pick up new coping skills, and gain a better comprehension of yourself.

Acknowledge Your Strengths: Don't allow depression to cast a shadow over your abilities.

Determine your strengths and the things that make you happy, then work on them.

Creating a Fulfilling Life: Find Your Passions: Get back involved in things you used to enjoy or take up new hobbies that make you happy and motivated.

Set Meaningful Goals: Achieving any size goal gives you a sense of purpose and success.

Foster Relationships: Social interaction is essential for overall health. Spend time fostering your relationships with family and friends and creating a network of people who can help you.

Give Back to Others: Giving back to others can increase one's sense of purpose and self-worth. Donate your time or expertise to a cause that is important to you.

Engage in Mindfulness Exercises: These can assist you in developing a calm attitude, focusing on appreciating the pleasant things in life in the here and now.

Adopt a Growth Mindset: Change your perspective so that obstacles are seen as chances to grow and learn.

Sustaining Well-Being:

Make self-care a priority. Emotional and physical health are based on getting enough sleep, eating a balanced diet, and exercising.

Handle Stress Well: Since stress can set off depressive episodes, learn healthy coping strategies to handle stress well.

Continue the Treatment: Even if you're feeling good, keep up with any prescribed therapy or medicine.

Honor Your Accomplishments: No matter how tiny, acknowledge and applaud your progress. This keeps you motivated and reinforces good conduct.

Seek Help When Needed: If you're having trouble, don't be afraid to ask for help from your therapist, relatives, friends, or support groups.

Living with Passion and Purpose: Leading a life full of passion, purpose, and connection is essential to thriving beyond depression.

Developing Resilience: You'll gain resilience as well as a better comprehension of your needs in terms of mental health.

Become an Inspiration: People going through difficult times may find encouragement in your story of recovery.

Rehab is a journey, not a destination, so keep that in mind. Along the route, there will be ups and downs. However, you may overcome depression and create a life that is meaningful, joyful, and well-being-filled with the correct resources and assistance.

You may create a life that flourishes and gets over depression by using these techniques and the tools that are out there. On this trip, you are not by yourself.

7.1. Developing Self-Esteem and Resilience

Self-worth and resilience are two potent psychological factors that combine to provide a solid basis for mental health. Here's how to foster both of them:

Recognizing the Relationship:

Self-Respect as the Basis: A strong feeling of self-worth supports your confidence in your capacity to overcome obstacles. You're more likely to overcome obstacles in life when you have confidence in yourself.

Resilience as the Shield: Resilience gives you the tools and abilities to get through challenging circumstances and come out stronger. It supports you in keeping an optimistic attitude amid hardship.

Developing Self-Respect:

Determine Your Advantages: Enumerate your abilities, aptitudes, and favorable attributes. Acknowledging your advantages increases confidence and self-belief.

Honor Your Accomplishments: Be proud of all of your achievements, no matter how modest. Recognize your efforts and advancement.

Preserve Treatment: Even if you're feeling well, stick to your doctor's recommendations for therapy or medicine.

Celebrate Your Accomplishments: No matter how tiny your progress may have been, acknowledge it. This keeps you motivated and reinforces good conduct.

Seek Help When Needed: If you're having trouble, don't be afraid to ask for help from your therapist, relatives, friends, or support groups.

Engage in Positive Self-Talk: Refute pessimistic ideas with empowering and realistic remarks about yourself. Pay attention to your abilities and capabilities.

Set Achievable Goals: As you achieve achievement, setting realistic goals will help you gain confidence. Honor accomplishments and draw lessons from failures.

Put Progress Before Perfection: Recognize that errors are unavoidable. Instead of concentrating on flaws, put your attention on growth and learning.

Establish Healthful Habits: Make a healthy diet, exercise, and sleep a priority. Having a positive self-image is correlated with physical well-being.

Accept Challenges: See obstacles as chances to improve and expand. Overcoming challenges increases resilience and self-worth. Developing Resilience

Create Well-Being Coping Strategies: To effectively handle difficult situations, acquire skills including emotional regulation, stress management, and relaxation techniques.

Establish a Robust Support Network: Be in the company of upbeat, encouraging individuals. overcoming obstacles.

<u>**Extra Advice**</u>:

Counseling: Take into account counseling to examine unfavorable self-perceptions and create more constructive coping strategies.

Support Groups: Make connections with people who are aware of the difficulties in developing resilience and self-worth.

Recall that developing resilience and self-worth is a continuous process. Celebrate your accomplishments, have patience with yourself, and don't be embarrassed to ask for help when you need it. By putting in the necessary time and effort, you may develop these essential traits and create a solid foundation for overcoming obstacles in life.

7.2. Positive Confession Therapy's (PCT) Effectiveness in

Treating Depression

PCT, or positive confession therapy, is a debatable method of treating depression. Although it has some appeal, there isn't any scientific evidence to support it, and it might even be detrimental. Here is a summary of its assertions and points to think about:

Core Principles of PCT:

Emphasis on Good Affirmations: PCT stresses substituting good ideas and beliefs for negative ones by repeating affirmations about oneself and one's future.

Religion-Based: Positive CBT, which suggests positive affirmations based on religion help heal depression, is frequently founded on religious principles.

Scripture can be a source of inspiration and consolation for those who are depressed. The following summarizes how religious literature can be used in addition to, but not as a substitute for, professional treatment:

Possible Help for Depression from Scripture:

Hope and Encouragement: A lot of the texts contain messages of God's love, hope, and perseverance, which can be comforting in trying times.

Sense of Community: For those who are depressed, religious communities can offer a solid support network and a sense of belonging.

Psalm 34:18: "The Lord is near to the brokenhearted and saves the crushed in spirit."

Isaiah 41:10: "Fear not, for I am with you; be not dismayed, for I am your God; I will strengthen you, I will help you, I will uphold you with my righteous right hand."

Matthew 11:28-30: "Come to me, all who labor and are heavily laden, and I will give you rest. Take my yoke upon you, and learn from me, for I am gentle and lowly in heart, and you will find rest for your souls. For my yoke is easy, and my burden is light."

Proverbs 3:5-6: "Trust in the Lord with all your heart, and lean not on your understanding. In all your ways acknowledge to him, and he shall direct your paths." (KJV) - This scripture emphasizes trusting in a higher power for guidance and strength, which can be a source of comfort during challenging times.

Philippians 4:13: "I can do all things through Christ who strengthens me." (KJV) - This verse reminds you that you are not alone and that with faith, you can overcome any obstacle, including depression.

Romans 8:28: "And we know that in all things God works for the good of those who love God and are called according to his purpose." (KJV) - This scripture offers hope and perspective, suggesting that even difficult times can ultimately lead to good.

2 Corinthians 12:9: "And he said unto me, **My grace is sufficient for thee**: for my strength is made perfect in weakness. Most gladly therefore will I rather glory in my infirmities, that the power of Christ may rest upon me." (KJV) - This verse reminds you that God's grace is enough, even in your moments of weakness. It can be a source of strength when facing depression.

Psalm 46:1: "God is our refuge and strength, a present help in time of need." (KJV) - This scripture offers a sense of security and comfort, knowing that God is always there to provide support during difficult times.

Jeremiah 29:11: "For I know the thoughts that I think toward you, saith the Lord, thoughts of peace, and not of evil, to give you an expected end." (KJV) - This verse offers hope for the future, reminding you that God has a plan for your life, even when you feel lost or hopeless.

1 John 4:18: "**There is no fear in love**, but perfect love casteth out fear: because fear hath torment. He that feareth is not made perfect in love.." (KJV)

- This scripture emphasizes the power of love to overcome fear, which can be a significant factor in depression.

It's critical to get professional assistance if you're depressed. While scripture can be a helpful ally on your road to recovery, it shouldn't take the role of

Positive Confessions' Possible Advantages:

Greater Attention to Positivity: Concentrating on uplifting statements may momentarily divert attention from unfavorable ideas.

Placebo impact: Having faith in the therapy may have a placebo impact, improving mood to some extent.

What Makes PCT a Contentious Issue?

Limited Scientific Evidence: The effectiveness of PCT in treating depression is not well-supported by scientific research.

Oversimplification of Depression: There are many contributing elements to depression, which is a complex disorder. The only focus of PCT on thinking modification might not address fundamental issues.

The Danger of Ignoring Underlying Problems: People who place too much emphasis on positive affirmations may downplay or deny deeper emotional problems that require attention.

Potential for Guilt: People may feel guilty or blame themselves if using positive affirmations doesn't result in a change in their symptoms right away.

Other Options for Depression Management:

Evidence-Based Therapies: Interpersonal therapy (IPT) and cognitive behavioral therapy (CBT) are highly helpful in treating depression and have substantial scientific support.

Medication: For certain patients, antidepressant medication may be an essential component of their treatment plan.

Lifestyle Adjustments: Making sleep, a good diet, and regular exercise a priority can greatly enhance mood and general well-being.

If you're experiencing depression, you should:

• Speak with a qualified mental health specialist who can evaluate your circumstances and provide a customized treatment plan based on therapies that are supported by research and address the underlying causes of your depression.

• A multitude of resources are accessible. to assist you in achieving your goal of recovery. Think about groups such as the Depression and Bipolar Support Alliance (DBSA) or the National Alliance on Mental Illness (NAMI).

Recall: There isn't a single treatment strategy for depression that works for everyone. Investigate your alternatives, give self-care priority, and get expert assistance for a successful and long-lasting recovery.

7.3 Discovering Intent and Goals

It can seem tough to find meaning and purpose when depression is present. The desire to interact with life might drastically decline when the world loses its liveliness. The good news is that meaning and purpose are still possible, even in the worst of depression. Here are a few methods for finding them again:

<u>**Changing the Way You See Things**</u>:

Pay Attention to Little Wins: Honor even your smallest successes. Taking a shower, finishing a task, or even just getting out of bed can be big victories in the fight against depression.

Change Your Perspective: Focus on the things you can still control rather than obsessing about the things you cannot. Perhaps it's taking in some quiet time in nature, reading a few chapters of a book, or listening to relaxing music.

Gratitude Practice: Make time every day to consider your blessings, no matter how minor. This can help you turn away from negativity and develop gratitude.

Linking Back to What's Important:

Go Back to Past Passions: Did you ever have a strong interest in performing, writing, or painting?

• Soundtrack? It could be intimidating, but think about taking up an old pastime again.

Investigate New Interests: Occasionally, learning something completely new ignites an idea. Examine several pursuits or volunteer opportunities to determine what piques your interest.

Put Your Attention on Helping Others: Even in

tiny ways, helping others can foster a feeling of connection and purpose. Give your time, lend a sympathetic ear to a friend, or carry out an act of spontaneous kindness.

Putting Together a Support Network:

Establish Contact with Family: Depression may intensify due to social isolation. Speak with a therapist, family member, or supportive friends for help. Talking about your difficulties can help you feel less alone and inspire you.

Support Groups: Making connections with people who are cognizant of depression can be immensely reassuring. Think about signing up for an online or local support group.

Recall that: The Journey Counts: Discovering meaning and purpose isn't about one big accomplishment at a time. It all comes down to the little measures you take every day to get ahead.

The Key Is Self-Compassion: Treat yourself with kindness. Healing is a journey, not a final destination. Despite the obstacles you may face, never give up on yourself.

Seek Professional Assistance: A therapist can help you find new meaning and purpose in your life as well as depression management techniques. Even in the face of depression's difficulties, you can progressively recover meaning and purpose in your life by implementing these measures and getting help. Recall that you are not alone and that there is hope.

7.4 Sustaining a State of Mental Well-Being:

Fostering a Life of Mental Well-Being Imagine living a life that gives you a sense of purpose, energy, and mastery. Where you can meet each day with serenity and hope and overcome obstacles with resiliency. This is how mental health can be powerful!

Being mentally well involves more than just not having any mental health issues. It involves deliberately fostering a condition of well-being that enables you to thrive in every area of your life. This is your manual for creating a thriving and colorful inner world:

Your Toolbox for Mental Wellness:

Meditation & Mindfulness: By practicing mindfulness and meditation, you can improve your focus and inner tranquility. Stress can be greatly reduced and emotional regulation can be enhanced by even a short daily session.

Make sleep a priority: Seize those Zzz's! Sleeping enough is essential for maintaining emotional and mental health. Aim for seven to eight hours of good sleep every night.

Feed Your Body: Your diet determines your health! Your body and brain are fueled for optimum mental health by a balanced diet high in fruits, vegetables, healthy grains, and lean meats.

Align Your Form: Fitness isn't the only aspect of exercise. Frequent exercise is a powerful way to reduce stress and improve mood. Discover your passions, whether it's dancing, swimming, working out at the gym, or taking brisk walks in the outdoors.

Embrace Positive Relationships: Be in the company of upbeat, encouraging people who elevate your spirits and make you feel wonderful. Having strong social ties is crucial for mental health.

Foster Gratitude: Make time every day to recognize and be grateful for all of life's blessings, no matter how minor Gratitude lessens negativity and promotes optimism.

Disprove Negative Thoughts: Thoughts have great power. Acquire the ability to recognize and confront unfavorable cognitive habits that may lead to psychological discomfort.

Employ Relaxation Techniques: Yoga, gradual muscle relaxation, and deep breathing exercises can all aid in stress reduction and the development of a calmer mindset.

Unplug and Recharge: It's important to take a break from technology and give yourself time to relax in this hyper-connected environment.

The Best Medicine Is Laughter: Laughing is a potent stress reducer and mood enhancer. Schedule time for the things that make you happy and laugh.

Customize Your Path to Wellbeing: This strategy is not one-size-fits-all. Try different things to see what suits you the best. Here are some pointers for making something unique:

• **Determine Your Stress Levels**: What makes you feel stressed out or fearful? Once you are aware, you can create coping strategies to deal with them successfully.

Locate Your Flow: What pursuits cause you to become engrossed in the here and now and lose sight of time? These are flow exercises, and they have a lot of mental health benefits.

Celebrate Little Wins: No matter how tiny, acknowledge and appreciate your accomplishments. This helps you stay inspired to continue on your wellness path by reinforcing beneficial actions.

Recall that mental health is a process rather than a destination. Along the route, there will be ups and downs. You can develop a robust and vibrant inner world by implementing these techniques and getting expert assistance as required. You have the right to a life of mental well-being!

CHAPTER 8

FREQUENTLY ASKED QUESTIONS AND ANSWERS ON DEPRESSION

Depression is a prevalent yet dangerous mental illness that can have a big impact on your attitude, ideas, and actions. The following are some responses to commonly posed questions concerning depression: What signs of depression are present? Depression symptoms might differ from person to person, however some typical ones are as follows:

• Losing interest in or enjoying activities you once enjoyed;

• Changing appetite or weight (weight gain or loss unrelated to dieting);

• Experiencing difficulty sleeping or sleeping too much;

• Experiencing feelings of guilt or worthlessness;

• Having trouble concentrating or making decisions; • Restlessness or feeling slowed down;

• Recurrent thoughts of death or suicide

What leads to depression?

Depression does not have a single cause. Several things may combine to cause it, such as:

Biological factors: Hormonal imbalances, genetics, and brain chemistry may all be relevant.

Psychological factors: Depression can be exacerbated by negative thought patterns, low self-esteem, and traumatic experiences in the past.

Stressors in life: Significant life events such as losing a job, having marital issues, or having financial troubles can set off depression. Is melancholy an indication of fragility? Not at all! Depression, like diabetes or heart disease, is a medical illness. It's not a reflection of weakness; it's just something you can't control. Is it possible to treat depression? Of course! One of the most easily treated mental health issues is depression.

There are primarily two types of care:

Medication: Antidepressant drugs can control mood-related chemicals in the brain.

Counseling: CBT, or cognitive behavioral therapy, is one other type of care for people with depression Meanwhile, both types of care when resorted to, can bring a faster recovery.

Finding Light After Darkness

Although depression can make you feel weighty, it doesn't have to define you. Here are 20 tales of tenacity, optimism, and depression recovery:

1. "I used to sleep all day, but now I wake up excited to paint." - Sarah, an artist: After struggling with melancholy for years, Sarah found comfort in art therapy and rediscovered her love of creating.

2. "The missing component was therapy. I can now at last control both my anxiety and my despair." - David, the instructor David battled anxiety and sadness, but treatment gave him the skills he needed to control both.

3. "Workout turned into my lifeline." It improved my quality of sleep and made me feel accomplished." - Author Emily: Emily learned how exercise may improve her emotions and found solace in a regular running schedule.

4. "My family became my support system." We were aware of one another's difficulties." Veteran Michael: After discovering he wasn't fighting

depression alone, Michael sought support and encouragement in a support group.

5. "Medication wasn't a cure, but it helped me feel well enough to start therapy." Student Jessica: Jessica accepted medicine as a first step toward treatment, realizing the value of both methods.

6. "Mindfulness meditation helped me quiet the negative thoughts." - Liam, a musician: Liam discovered inner peace by using mindfulness techniques to control his negative thoughts.

7. "I had to learn to say no and prioritize my well-being." - Olivia, an entrepreneur: Olivia's stress and depressive symptoms decreased when she learned to prioritize self-care and set limits. Forgiveness of oneself was essential. Depression wasn't a result of me." - Noah, Therapist: Acquiring self-compassion enabled Noah to let go of self-blame, which was a crucial component of his rehabilitation.

9. "Volunteering helped me find purpose again." - Sophia, a nurse: Volunteering gave Sophia a sense of purpose and community, which was a great way to fight sadness.

10. "My dog served as my furry counselor. I had a cause to get out of bed thanks to him." - Ethan, IT specialist: Ethan learned the comfort and emotional support a pet can provide in trying times.

11. "Reading self-help books opened my eyes to new perspectives." - Chloe, a graphic designer: By reading self-help books, Chloe gained insight and resilience and discovered new coping mechanisms for depression.

12. "Connecting with nature helped me feel grounded." Daniel, the chef: Being outside has become a source of serenity and relaxation reducing the symptoms of depression for Daniel.

13. "Healthy eating fueled my body and mind." - Mia, Teacher: Mia adopted a healthy diet after seeing the link between a person's physical and mental health.

14. "Learning to say 'thank you' shifted my focus to gratitude." Engineer William: By cultivating gratitude, William was able to lessen the negativity that comes with depression and adopt a more upbeat perspective.

15. "Deep breathing exercises became my go-to stress relief tool." - Ava, Artist: Ava employs basic breathing techniques regularly to manage her anxiety and stress.

16. "Journaling allowed me to express my emotions and gain clarity." - Lucas, Student: Journaling gave Lucas a secure place to talk about his emotions and monitor his healing process.

17. "Music listening improved my mood and assisted me handling your feelings." - Amelia, a musician: Amelia used music as a coping method for her depression since it provided her with emotional release and solace.

18. "Spending time with loved ones reminded me I wasn't alone." - Benjamin, Architect: Reminding himself of his support network, Benjamin made bolstering his social ties a top priority.

19. "Learning to say 'no' helped me prioritize my needs." - Social worker Charlotte: Charlotte was able to take charge of her recovery by putting her own needs first and establishing healthy boundaries.

20. "Healing isn't a straight line. Even when I have good and terrible days, I never stop trying." - Matthew, Author: Although he recognized the difficulties in healing, Matthew highlighted the value of tenacity and hope.

<u>REFERENCES</u>

The following further materials might be useful to you:

- Depression and Bipolar Support Alliance (DBSA): https://www.dbsalliance.org/

- National Alliance on Mental Illness (NAMI): https://www.nami.org/

- MentalHealth.gov: https://www.samhsa.gov/mental-health

- The Jed Foundation: https://www.jedfoundation.org/ (Focuses on mental health resources for teens and young adults)

- Depression and Bipolar Support Alliance (DBSA): https://www.dbsalliance.org/ MentalHealth.gov: https://www.samhsa.gov/mental-health

Technology can be a powerful tool for enhancing mental wellness. Here are some resources to explore:

- **Headspace:** https://www.headspace.com/ (Guided meditations)

- **Calm:** https://www.calm.com/ (Meditation, sleep stories, and relaxation techniques)

- **Happify:** https://www.happify.com/ (Science-backed activities to improve mood)